Natural Detox Cleanse Guide for Health

Using Diet Plans to Lose Weight the Right Way

By: Barry Short

I0121887

PUBLISHERS NOTES

Disclaimer

This publication is intended to provide helpful and informative material. It is not intended to diagnose, treat, cure, or prevent any health problem or condition, nor is intended to replace the advice of a physician. No action should be taken solely on the contents of this book. Always consult your physician or qualified health-care professional on any matters regarding your health and before adopting any suggestions in this book or drawing inferences from it.

The author and publisher specifically disclaim all responsibility for any liability, loss or risk, personal or otherwise, which is incurred as a consequence, directly or indirectly, from the use or application of any contents of this book.

Any and all product names referenced within this book are the trademarks of their respective owners. None of these owners have sponsored, authorized, endorsed, or approved this book.

Always read all information provided by the manufacturers' product labels before using their products. The author and publisher are not responsible for claims made by manufacturers.

Paperback Edition

Manufactured in the United States of America

Barry Short

DEDICATION

I thank my wife Emma for showing me how a detox can help to get the rest that it needs. We push our bodies pretty hard on a daily basis and when we eat healthily we blow it out of the water.

TABLE OF CONTENTS

CHAPTER 1- HOW TO ACHIEVE A SUCCESSFUL NATURAL DETOX

Natural Detox regimens have been increasing in popularity for several years. With so many pollutants in the air we breathe and the environment we live in it is likely that awareness of Natural detox will continue to grow in the coming years. Detox is the process of removing toxins from the body.

Whether toxins were inhaled, injected or consumed they tend to stay in the body – often in fatty tissue.

So we cannot just hope to flush the toxins away by drinking a lot of pure water. If only it was so easy to detoxify the body – we would all be a lot healthier and happier.

Natural detox means that we use natural detox supplements and natural detox aids such as a skin brush or maybe an enema kit to help us and not pharmacy drugs which could add to the burden to toxins in the body already.

We need to take a smart approach to detox – one that works with the body's natural process of detoxification. We do this in several ways...O did I tell you that detox may take several months? It all depends on the toxins you are working on and the state of your health at the time of the detox.

Yes you can follow a detox program for a week or so and it will benefit you if it is well designed but a thorough natural detox will take as many months as it takes the body to process and eliminate the toxins.

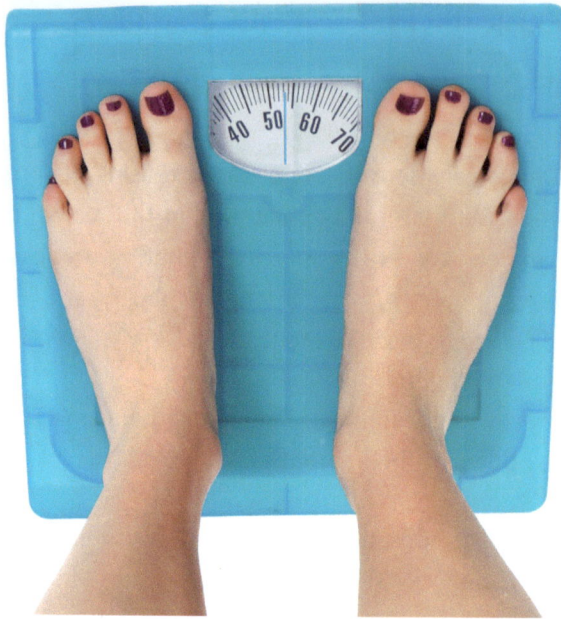

General advice is to get healthy as you can before attempting to detox and to follow proper professional guidance of a well qualified detox expert such as a Naturopathic Doctor.

See the Whole Picture by Taking a Holistic Approach

A holistic detox will take place at a speed that you can handle comfortably. Detox is a stress on you and if you are stressed already you need to pace the detox in line with your strength and ability to cope.

Take the Detox Step By Step

You have a whole body to detox so where do you start? There are 3 major body systems involved in your body detox and we focus on them one after the other to make it as easy as possible to do a proper detox and have as few detox symptoms as possible. My approach is to start with some general detox techniques such as skin brushing and saunas to get the process started in a gentle way. Then we start system by system...

Start With the Colon

There is a saying that we should start with the end in mind! Never was that more true than in natural detox. Colon cleansing is the first major part of the detox puzzle. This is a pretty easy process and can be done without changing your routine all that much. You may want to spend a month on this stage. Naturally as you detox the colon you'll be following a clean healthy diet with as much fresh salads and vegetables as possible.

Continue With a Kidney Detox

The second major stage of a natural detox is to follow a good kidney detox. There are several natural detox supplements to support the kidneys and there are many kidney cleansing herbs. Take it easy and take a month and as I said above take professional advice too.

Natural Detox Tip: we get to the liver!

The liver is the most serious and dedicated detox organ in the body and we need to prepare the body properly before we start to do liver cleansing or liver detox. Again there are several super liver detox nutrients and supplements and liver detox herbs too.

A clean diet including alcohol avoidance is important when detoxing the liver. As the natural detox tips above are followed the body will feel more energetic and yes you may get some healing side effects. You may get headaches or rashes breaking out on the skin.

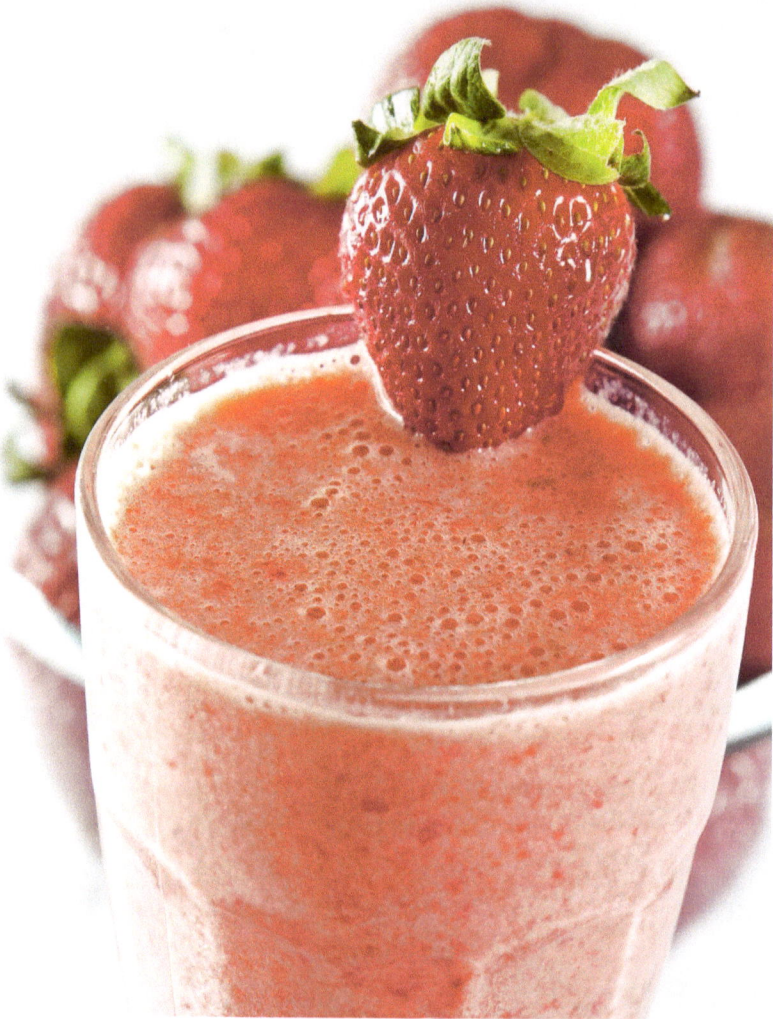

This is why it is best to detox with a Naturopath helping you. After the detox you will likely sleep better, feel more energetic and have clearer skin. There are many benefits of going through a natural detox. If you care about keeping healthy and are willing to put in

Barry Short

the effort then the natural detox tips above will help you achieve better health and lead a happier and fuller life.

CHAPTER 2- WHY DO A DAILY DETOX?

Daily detox is an idea that sounds a little strange until you realize that we are breathing drinking and eating toxins daily so why not help the body detox daily?

There are several ways to do this. At the heart of it we need to build awareness of the toxic environment we live in and be willing to adjust to the need of the body for clean water, organic food and clean air.

Taking a well designed daily detox formula helps too.

Some people like to take a daily detox clay formula. I don't usually recommend using clay orally but there can be special reasons for doing a short term cleanse using clay.

More often a good detox blend of herbs is used. Because you are taking these daily the doses needs to be right. Detox herbs are usually taken once or twice a year in a change of the seasons type detox and cleanse program. Taking these herbs daily could in principle cause a problem so the doses need to be small enough for daily use.

Typical of such daily detox blends would be herbs such as milk thistle, artichoke leaf, dandelion leaf, marshmallow root, red clover and slippery elm.

How to Take the Daily Detox?

Usually you can find blends to take as a tea – which is my favorite way or as a tincture or capsule which are both very easy to take and very convenient. A tincture or capsule may be best for a child since teas are often rather strong or have a bitter taste even if you do use honey to disguise it.

Please be careful about dosage for a child because the correct dose depends on the age of the child. Children can safely detox but gentle blends of herbs should be used and it is best to have professional help in such cases.

How to Take the Daily Detox?

Usually you can find blends to take as a tea – which is my favorite way or as a tincture or capsule which are both very easy to take and very convenient.

A tincture or capsule may be best for a child since teas are often rather strong or have a bitter taste even if you do use honey to disguise it. Please be careful about dosage for a child because the correct dose depends on the age of the child. Children can safely detox but gentle blends of herbs should be used and it is best to have professional help in such cases.

Five Foods to Have Before the Detox

The hardest part for most dieters is having to restrict or eliminate some of their favorite foods from their diet. It is unfortunate that delicious foods are often unhealthy. However, some of these so-called unhealthy foods are actually quite nutritious, and it would be a shame to exclude them from your diet based on misconceptions.

Chili

Most people picture chili as an unhealthy food due to its association with fattening fast food dishes like chili dogs and chili cheese fries. It may surprise you to know that chili boasts a robust profile of nutrients. The meat provides protein while the tomatoes, peppers, and onions contribute numerous vitamins and minerals. Beans will add even more protein plus Vitamin B6, iron, riboflavin, and more. Be sure to use lean meat to keep the fat content down.

Ask your butcher for ground round or ground sirloin; these are the leanest cuts of ground beef. Using ground turkey is another healthy option. If you top your chili with cheese or sour cream, use them in moderation.

Steak

Steak is often eschewed by dieters in favor of white meat or seafood, but a thick slab of red meat can be more nutritious than commonly thought.

Steak has a very high density of protein per ounce, helping dieters build muscle and stay full after meals. The leanest cuts of steak are sirloin and top round. The most popular way to cook a steak happens to be the healthiest as well: over red-hot coals.

Grilling forms a delicious browned crust on the meat and allows excess fat to drip off. If you do not have a barbecue grill or the weather is an impediment, invest in a cast iron grill pan for similar results.

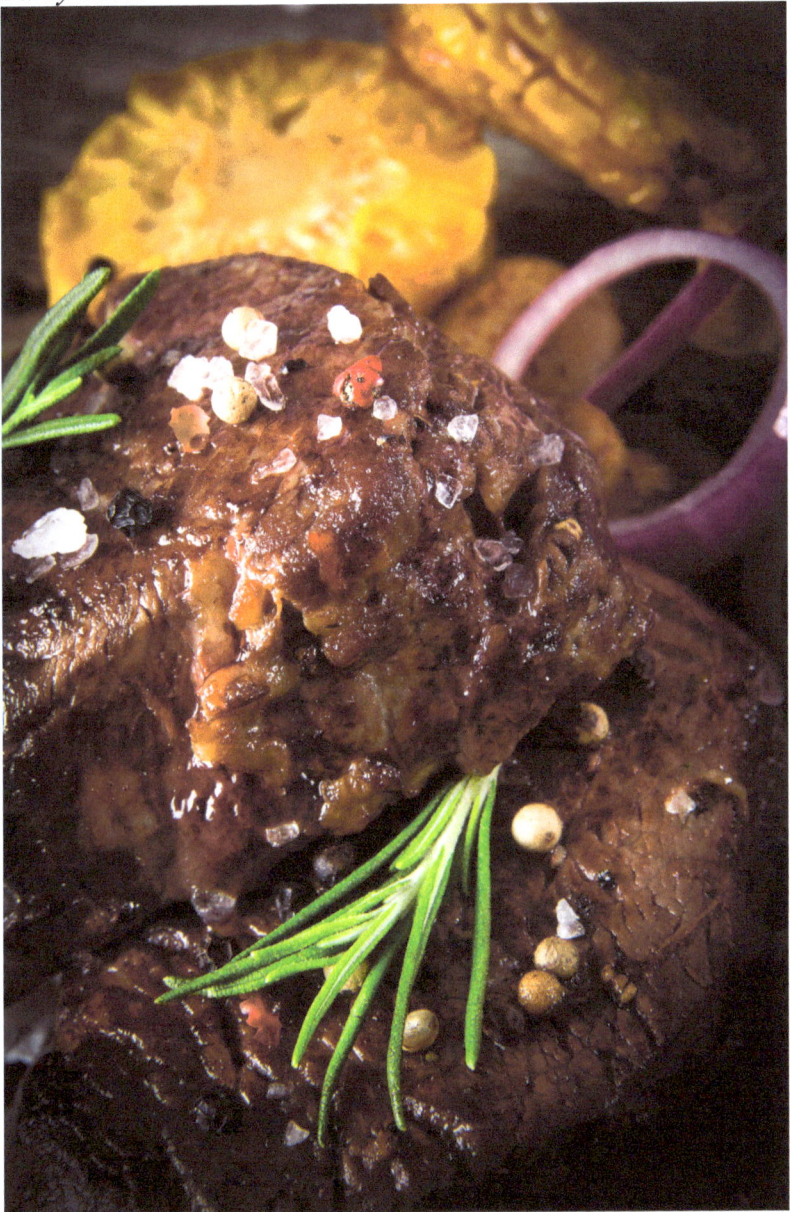

Shrimp

This diminutive sea creature has developed a reputation as an indulgence food. The problem is that shrimp is usually deep-fried or smothered in fatty cream sauces.

Familiarizing yourself with some healthy shrimp recipes will allow you to enjoy this seafood while staying focused on your fitness goals. Shrimp is excellent when soaked in marinade and grilled on skewers. Cooked shrimp are delicious on top of a green salad as well. Even the classic shrimp cocktail is fairly nutritious. Just remember to go easy on the cocktail sauce; it contains a large amount of sodium.

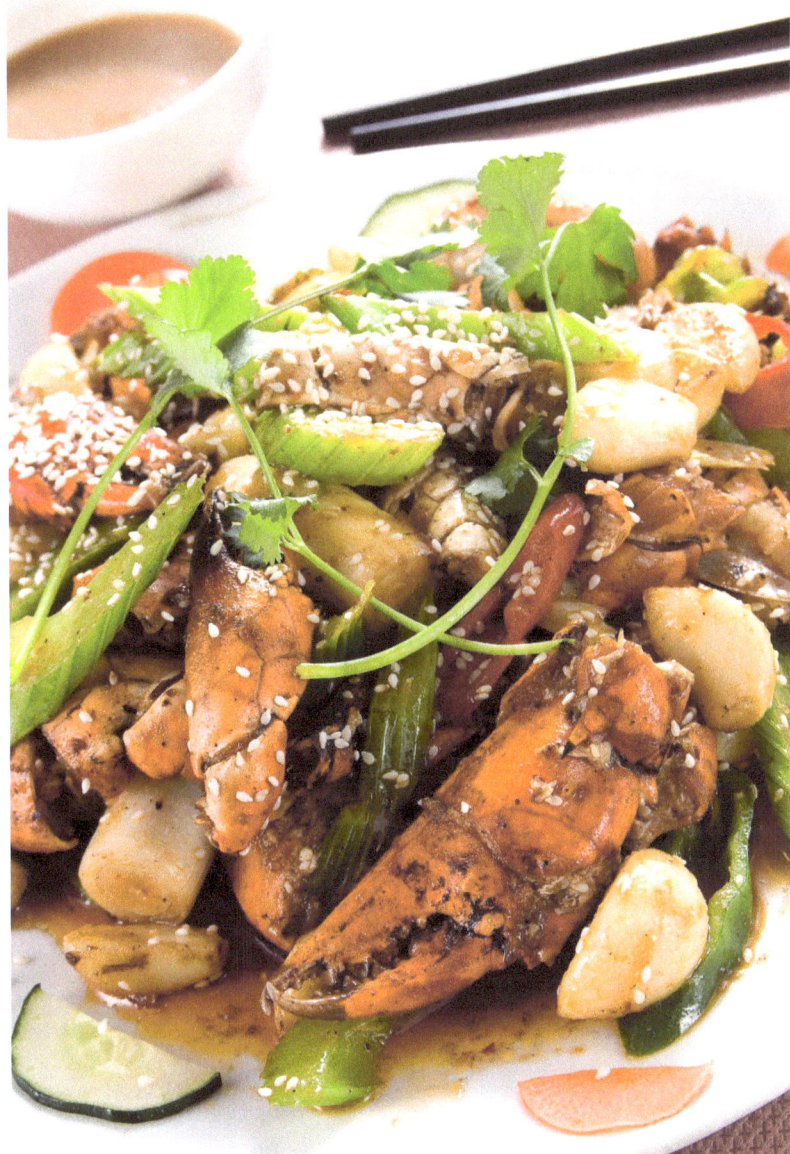

Stir-fry

Keep in mind that the stir-fry dishes you'll find at a Chinese buffet are indeed unhealthy. They tend to use excessive amounts of lard and sugary sauces. This is unfortunate because stir-frying can produce some very healthy meals.

The advantage of stir-fry cooking is that it can effectively fry a large amount of food with a small amount of oil. A very nutritious meal can be made by stir-frying fresh vegetables with lean meats. Broccoli pairs well with almost any meat; consider stir-frying it with some of the previously mentioned shrimp or steak.

Towards the end of the cooking process, you can give the dish an exotic Far Eastern flavor by adding garlic, ginger, and a few dashes of soy sauce and sweet rice wine. But stir-frying is not limited to Asian cuisine - dishes like ratatouille are excellent when cooked in a wok.

Eggs

Some dieticians demonize eggs due to the saturated fat and cholesterol content. These substances may be present in eggs, but a few eggs per day is not going to put anyone at risk for heart problems.

Furthermore, research has shown that ingesting cholesterol does not contribute to the levels of cholesterol in the blood. The great thing about eggs is the endless number of ways to cook them. Omelets, frittatas, or scrambled eggs all make a great breakfast. They can also be hard-boiled and enjoyed as a convenient snack.

Keep in mind that a food is not necessarily unhealthy just because it is frequently prepared in unhealthy ways. Look at the nutritional value of the ingredients and you may find that a certain food is healthier than you previously believed.

Continuing to enjoy these delicious foods in nutritious ways will make it easier and more enjoyable to stick to your diet.

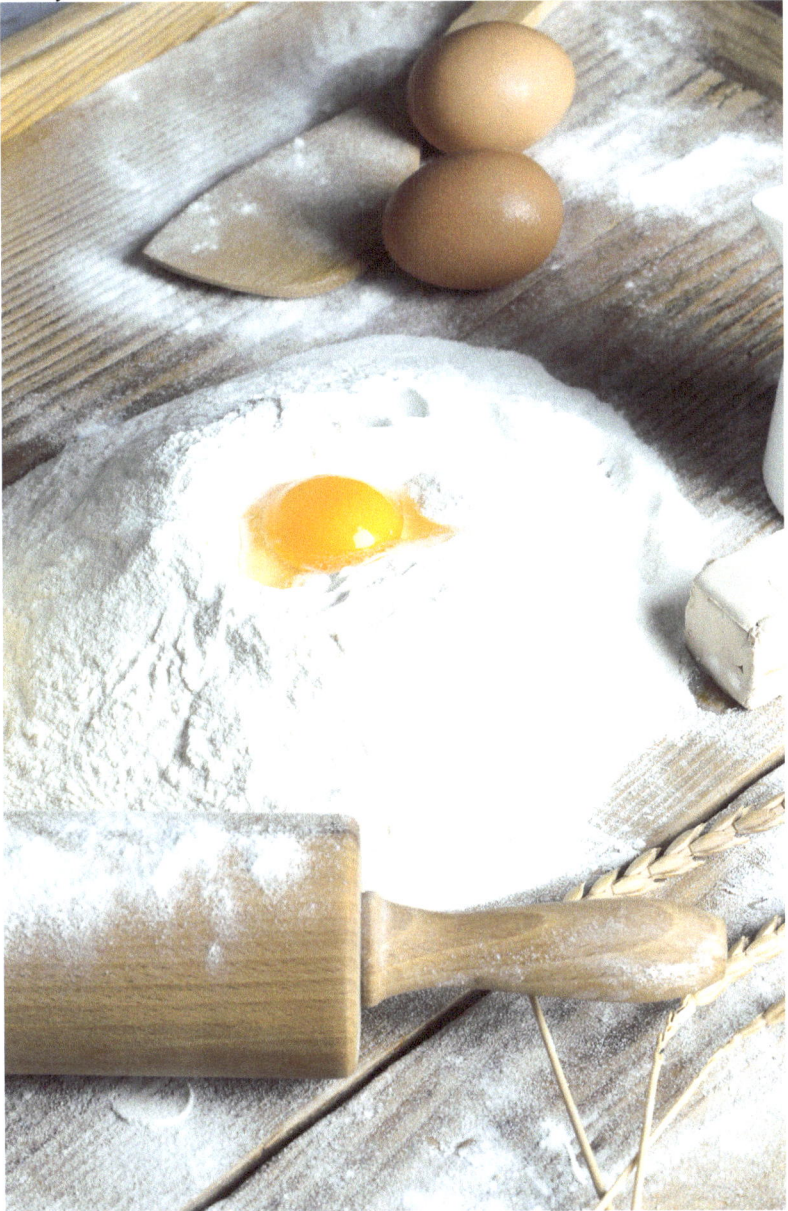

CHAPTER 3- DETOXING THE KIDNEY

Of the 3 stages of a thorough detox – *colon cleansing, kidney detox and liver detox the kidney detox is the least popular*.

This is strange really because the kidneys get the brunt of all the toxins in the blood hitting them so they need support to do their job efficiently.

Of the many functions of the kidneys we'll focus on detox and at the simplest level we can think of the kidneys as being filters for the blood.

They excrete waste products like ammonium and urea and work hard to purify the blood – the filtration is not passive like a coffee filter but active and needs a lot of energy to keep it going.

A toxic blood stream is going to expose the tissues of the kidney to damage and impose a healing burden on the rest of the body.

That gives us an idea on why we need kidney detox now we take a look at how we go about this.

First of all any toxins removed by the kidney will end up in the bladder so a major part of any kidney detox must be to support the bladder.

This is why along with traditional kidney and bladder herbs I recommend using a gram or two of vitamin C per day.

The vitamin C will wash through the blood stream and kidney and some of it will flush out the ureters leading from the kidney to the bladder and be collected in the bladder. Having the gentle protective effect of extra vitamin C makes a lot of sense with or without a detox.

Standard kidney herbs include our old friend dandelion and soothing corn silk and horsetail. An all round herb for the urinary system is bearberry also known as Uva Ursi.

These can be taken as a tincture which makes taking the detox herbs very easy and that makes it more likely that we will stick to it for the duration of the detox program.

These detox herbs can be used as part of an overall kidney detox along with a detox diet and professional help! They are not supposed to treat or dissolve or expel kidney stones – that is a serious issue needing personal consultation.

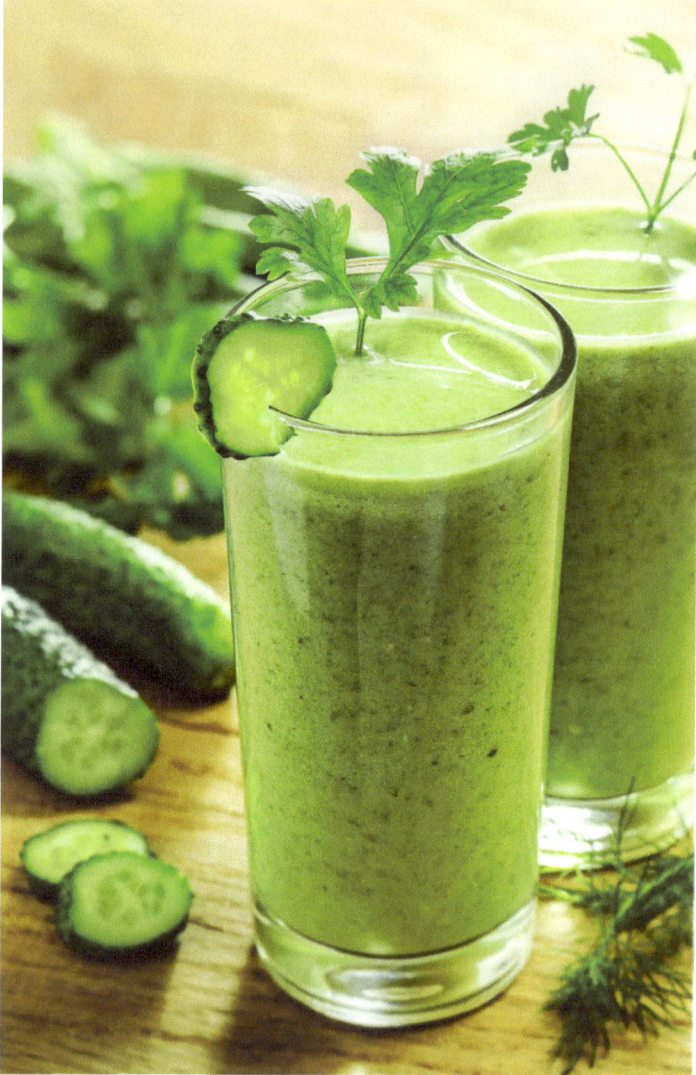

CHAPTER 4- THE DETOX FOOT PATCH

Is a Detox Foot Patch the easy way to detox? Some people think so and you can read their testimonials. But slapping a foot patch on the soles of your feet overnight seems effortlessly easy and rather unlikely as a detox technique.

But this is something we would all love to be effective!

After all who wants to drink green juices for months or mix psyllium husks with water as part of a colon cleanse or take our Milk Thistle and Dandelion herbal teas and tinctures if all we needed to do was...go to sleep with a foot patch on and wake up detoxed!

So What's Going On?

Detox foot patches are not a recent fad. They have been around for 4 years at least and are not to be confused with the foot pads used by Podiatrists and Chiropractors when they are working to support humdrum problems like fallen arches and sub optimal gait.

Detox Foot Patches and Pads Are Different

There are several brands of detox foot patch - Kinoki, Chikusaku, Takara to name a few. All are claiming that the pads or patches detox the body but where is the proof they claim to have?

Scientific claims that I cannot check or verify in some way are simply not believable.

A few years ago some scientists made claims that energy was being produced by a battery cell device they constructed and that the energy produced was nuclear energy. This claim that "cold nuclear fusion" was occurring caused a huge ruckus and many experimental groups tried to check the results. After a while it seemed that the whole thing was hoopla. No results could be found to support the claims.

My position is that it is fine to talk about detox and traditional Chinese or Oriental medicine but when push comes to shove there is no proof for detox by foot pad and we are all left looking at testimonials and wondering if there is anything real.

Detox is a real and valid set of procedures to eliminate toxins from the liver and from the fat cells of your body and all this can be measured and verified.

If health claims are made but not backed up and no proof is forth coming even after multiple challenges then we can just get on with the rest of our day.

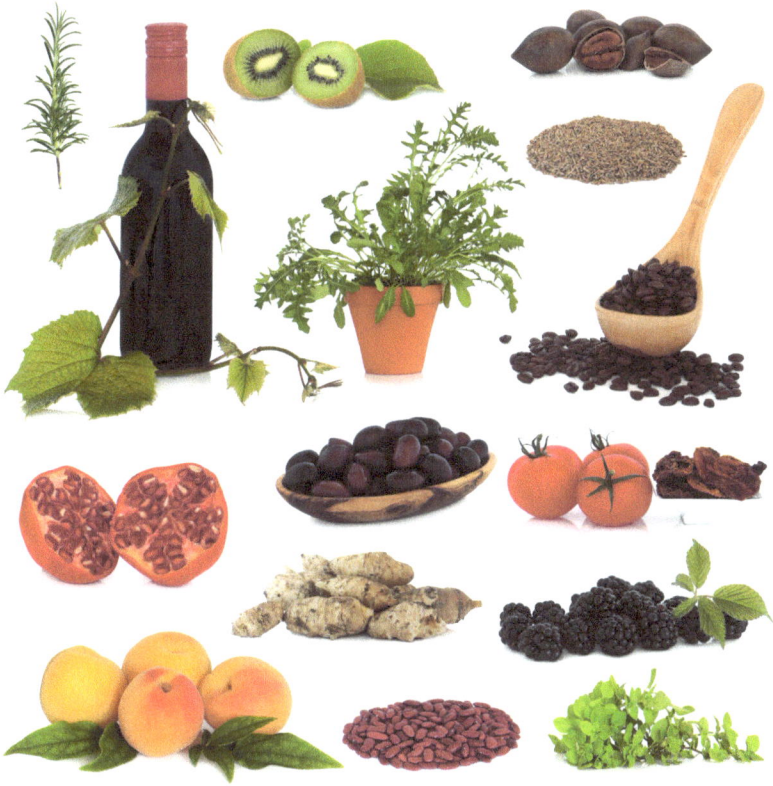

Unless I can see some scientific experimental laboratory proof I'll regard detox foot patches as "pending validation" at best and an outright scam at worst.

PS Putting herbal and other medical ingredients on a cloth / patch / pad is what a poultice is and people have been using herbal poultices for centuries. Suppose we just forget the word "detox" here and regard these foot patches in the same way we look at foot baths and other topical treatments?

We may find that some of these "foot poultices" have genuine therapeutic effect and an effect that is not connected to detox at all.

CHAPTER 5- WHO IS ON A DETOX DRIVE?

I was browsing as you do on the Net – with no particular thing to do. I noticed on a Detox blog that shall remain nameless, an idiotic post that got me smacking my forehead and asking, and "Who writes this stuff?"

Here were some of the gems of gleaming wisdom I gleaned there:

Drink 8 Glasses of Water Daily

Not only is there not the slightest shred of scientific backup for this there is even research into this silliness which shows just how unfounded it is.

If this was based on real science we would find discussions and arguments for various amounts of water. There would be allowances for climate, age of the person concerned as well as their weight.

Scientists from different disciplines would be giving different advice.

Getting scientists to agree on one number is hard and for them to come up with a neat not to say cute rule like 8 glasses a day or 8 Oz glasses a day is about as likely as winning the lottery 8 days in a row!

Eat Lots of Colorful Food

The last time I looked burgers, fries and coke all had color. I am being a tad sarcastic here because I know what they are aiming at.

The advice refers to including a variety of different salads and fruits when you detox.

Your diet while you detox is important. It can either get in the way – which is what the burger, fries and soda diet would do or help a little which is what a diet rich in superfoods would do. The color though is not the issue; the issue is the quality and freshness of the food.

Drop the Caffeine

If you are a coffee addict then cutting back to one or none may well give you a hard time. It is best to prepare for a Detox by gradually cleaning up your diet over the previous days and even weeks. There's no need to put yourself through a hard time when you can avoid it.

Green tea has caffeine and is a superfood so caffeine should not be confused with "coffee addict". Other tea has caffeine too although much less than coffee.

Definitely avoid caffeine drinks in the evening though because they may well make it harder to relax and get to sleep.

Natural Detox Cleanse

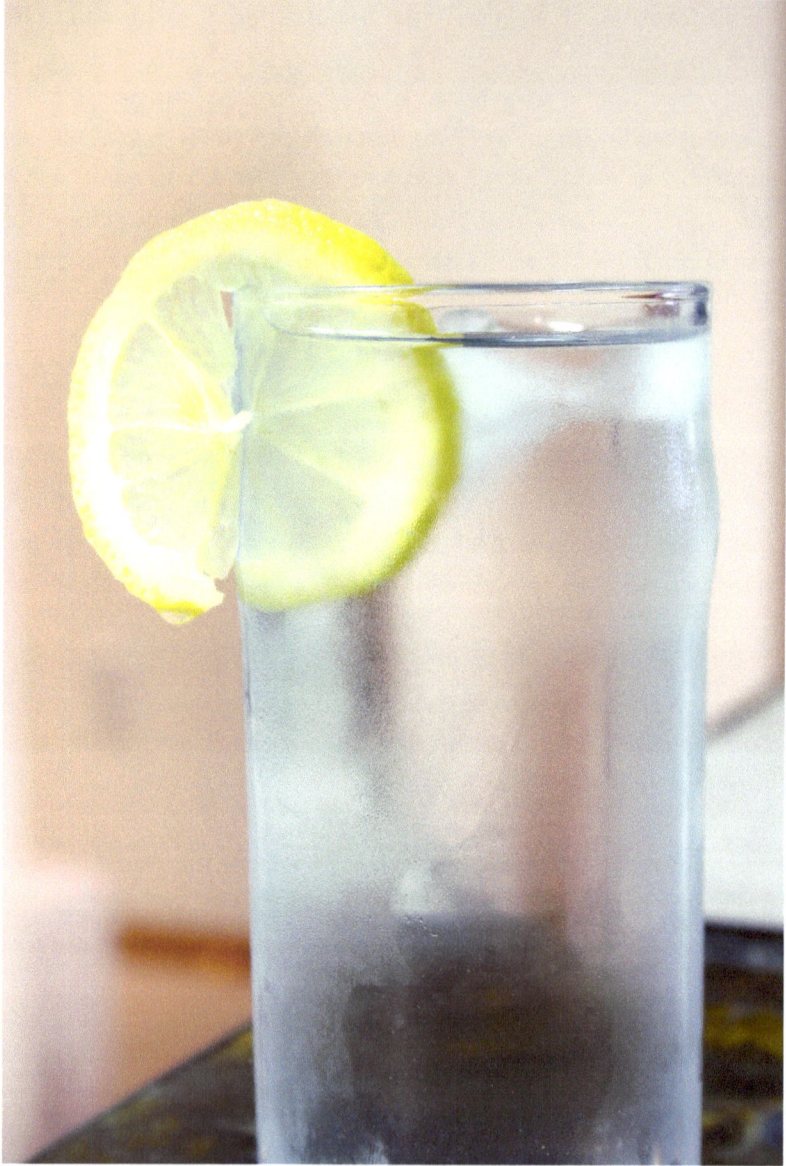

CHAPTER 6- WHAT OF THE FRUIT DETOX?

Detox plans may differ a lot. The detox supplements differ with some being herbal and others amino acid based. The diets to support the detox vary widely as well. You may be advised to follow rice based macrobiotic diet or to use a fruit detox diet.

Fruit, and that would be organic fruit, has many advantages for anyone following a detox plan. Fruit is usually sweet and we all love sweet things. Often it is the overconsumption of starchy sweet foods that lead to the weight gain or health problem that is responsible for your detox.

Fruit requires little preparation. You may be feeling run down and the last thing you want to do is spend hours cooking.

Fruit is easy to consume and leaves you feeling satisfied – you've had a sweet fix without any guilt so that all sounds good.

Fruit Detox Plan

A Fruit Detox has to be planned just like any other detox plan. You need to do the right shopping to get enough fruit to cover you for the period of your detox. Mostly a fruit detox would take a weekend or a few days and consists only of fruit and pure water.

I guess we can stretch a point and allow you some fruit teas as well!

Often the day starts with some lemon in hot water and then followed up with some crunchy fruit like apples that satisfy the need many people have to bite and chew. Some fruit detox plans include starchy fruit like bananas others advise against them. For sure, fruit juice is best avoided because it will just give you a sugar high and then dump you in a sugar low or hypoglycemic low energy period.

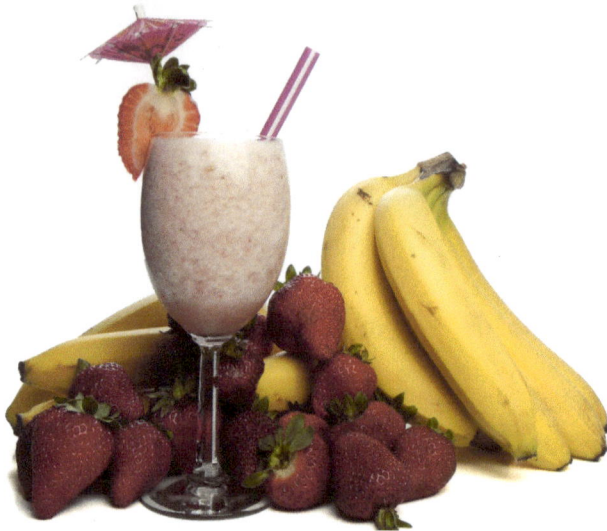

People with diabetes or who are hypoglycemic are strongly advised to consult with a health professional before taking this kind of detox. In my view this is not the kind of detox plan that suits those with blood sugar issues.

Otherwise a fruit detox diet is fine for a day or so – why not organize a few friends and make it an event to look forward to?

The fruits and vegetable diet is ideal for people who seek to lose some excessive pounds, get a boost in nutrition that they missed in other meals, and also enjoy new tastes that only natural foods have.

In fact, having vegetables and fruits, and absolutely no meat, for the three daily meals is possible and at the same time sensible. It is also worth noting that an organic or natural meal can be prepared with much less time, energy and effort when compared to preparing meat dishes or fried foods.

As such, a fruit and vegetable diet is recommended for people who are too busy at work and have not much time left to take care of their wellness. No time to exercise during the work week?

Getting used to those convenient but unhealthy foods served at joints like McDonald's, Krispy Kreme and Baskin Robbins? It's time to start a new strategy that can lead to a healthier lifestyle.

A fruits and vegetable diet can be a new and good way to enjoy meals during the week. If anyone feels that such a diet may be too drastic for them to adjust with, he or she can adapt it for as short as two days and then return to the old ways. On the first day, one can replace the usual eggs, ham, toasted bread and coffee breakfast with a new one composed of a slice of whole wheat bread, a cup of broccoli, a fresh fruit (an apple), and a single serving of green tea in a cup or a simple glass of water. Instead of having steak, mashed potato and soda for lunch, a set of cream mushroom soup, a garden salad (with lettuce, carrots, cucumbers, broccoli, olives and shredded cheese), a piece of banana and a glass of orange juice is recommended.

For dinner, the dieter can have Caesar salad, a cup of vanilla ice cream, one or two small fruits (either apples or oranges) and water.

For the next day, a bowl of oatmeal, a piece of banana (or a bowl of strawberries if bananas are not available), a few soda crackers and a cup of green tea or a glass of grapefruit juice is nice to start the day.

At lunch, one can have a veggie burger as the main course along with a bowl of corn soup, a cup of stuffed mushrooms, a cup of mango slices and a glass of water can be sufficient to last the rest of the day. At home, dinner can be composed of a veggie pizza, a slice of pumpkin cake, a cup of strawberries, a cup of vanilla ice cream and a glass of fruit juice or water.

By the end of two days, the dieter's metabolism should be faster, more nutrients should have been absorbed and a few pounds could have been lost.

To really implement the fruits and vegetable diet on a schedule for the short term, one must consult with either a nutritionist or a physician for guidance. At the very least, the meals suggested here should prove not only healthy to busy people but also more convenient to prepare and less expensive to deal with. Time and money saved from the exclusion of meat or fatty foods will easily be noticed.

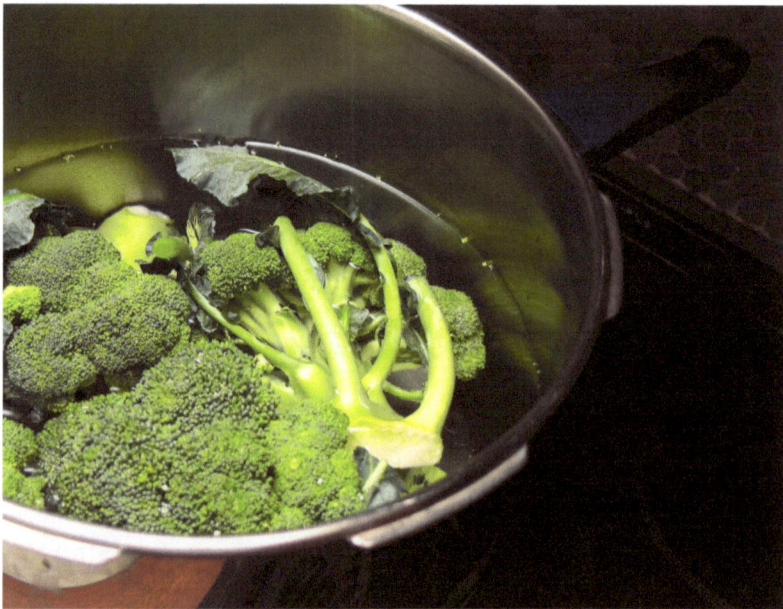

CHAPTER 7- DETOX TEA ANYONE?

Detoxing is a great way to improve your health and a great way to learn about how much good you can do for yourself. It's great to get expert advice on health when you need it and a thorough detox is one of those times but using a good detox tea as part of the daily routine is a nice and easy health measure that takes little effort.

Detox teas are easy to make and many are delicious too. Most are blends of herbs chosen for their ability to work with each other and blend not just their detox ability but their taste too.

One nice example is liquorice. Liquorice is one of the most important herbs in Oriental Medicine and plays a big role in many herbal formulas. The sweet taste and neutral energy and adrenal support help a detox tea by giving a great taste and a mild laxative action.

Traditional detox teas are made from herbs such as dandelion, milk thistle and nettles – all of which are regarded by gardeners as weeds. All of which are known to herbalists and Naturopaths as useful detox herbs that can be prepared to make a detox tea.

If you have an herb shop available then you can just buy fresh herbs and prepare them in your kitchen whenever you like.

Of course many are widely available and you can pick them and use them with the permission of the landowner. The problem with that is of identification! Unless you are an expert or have had personal training it is all too easy to pick the wrong plant!

When you buy a detox herb from herbal suppliers there is little chance of such mistakes. Usually they will source the herbs from a dedicated herb farm and not from wild craft.

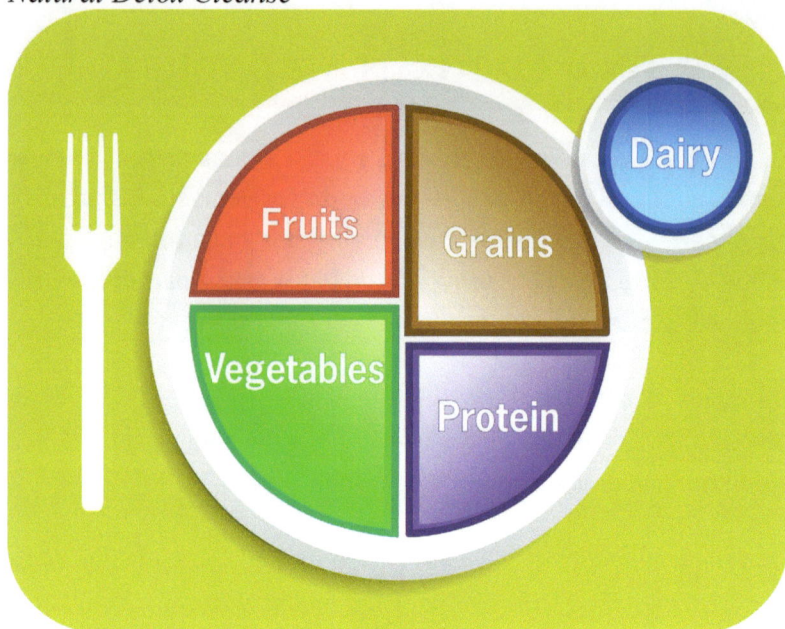

And of course you can make a delicious detox tea just using a teabag. I start my day with a big cup of licorice also spelt liquorice tea and find it calming and invigorating.

Using detox teas as part of a daily routine can help you deal with the toxins from the environment and make any detox program you follow easier for you because you will be doing a little detox every day.

Detoxing is a great way to improve your health and a great way to learn about how much good you can do for yourself.

It's great to get expert advice on health when you need it and a thorough detox is one of those times but using a good detox tea as part of the daily routine is a nice and easy health measure that takes little effort.

CHAPTER 8- CHOCOLATE, A SUPERFOOD?

Chocolate is one of the most desirable of all foods. It is a traditional gift at Mother's day and often a gift made by men to try to compensate for an act of thoughtlessness.

Why Chocolate Is Called the "Food of the Gods"?

The chocolate tree, Theobroma Cacao, has been grown in Central, South America and Mexico for centuries but only known in Europe since Cortes and Columbus.

The chocolate and cocoa that we know is quite different from the creations that Aztec and Mayans prepared. It had a central role in the religious ceremonies of the time and the name of the tree Theobroma Broma ("food of the Gods.")

Does Chocolate Really Grow on Trees?

Sort of! What really grows on trees are the cocoa pods which contain the cocoa beans. After a complicated process involving roasting, crushing and fermentation we get the chocolate. And in Europe the dark taste of what I always call "real chocolate" was masked with sugar amongst other things!

Which Type of Chocolate?

The picture above shows dark chocolate, milk chocolate and white chocolate and all have healthy effects but the scientific research is focused on dark chocolate because it has higher amounts of natural polyphenols.

Dark chocolate has a bitter taste because it is not mixed in with all the extra fat and sugar that are in the standard chocolate bars.

Research has shown health effects of eating even a slim amount of real chocolate in a number of different ways ...

Reduction of plaque on the inside of arteries

Reduction of oxidation of LDL cholesterol

Reduction of risk from stroke

Coughs are suppressed more effectively than by codeine

Anti-diarrhea effect

Increase of insulin sensitivity

High magnesium food helps with relaxation

Looking at these health effects as well as the desirability and palatability of chocolate we can see that chocolate is a superfood that we can eat often with great benefit.

The only caveat is that the superfood we speak of here is the Dark Chocolate and not the "Candy chocolate" that is a high fat and high sugar item found in stores worldwide.

<u>That is junk food and not at all the food of the Gods!</u>

CHAPTER 9- THE SEVEN DAY DETOX PLAN

Can You Do a Detox in 7 Days?

Well it all depends on your expectations. You cannot remove all the toxins from your body in 7 days – or 7 weeks for that matter. Many toxins are deep in our tissues – fatty tissues or even in our bones and would take months of detoxing to remove.

But you can do some good detoxing in a week and resume the process any time you choose.

First Step – Getting Clear

Let's be clear first what detox is and what it is not. There are tons of websites and magazine mindlessly babbling about detox and this causes much confusion.

Detox is not about dieting, slimming or weight loss. It is a vital part of building your health and has been used in East and West for centuries. The purpose is to prepare yourself for a healthier future.

Second Step – The Detox Diet

A Detox diet is a part of all detox programs. It will typically be rich in fruit and vegetables, be easy to digest and devoid of foods which are allergenic to the individual.

The food chosen may vary a lot depending on what kind of meals you prefer but the emphasis is on fresh and organic produce. If you eat foods that have been sprayed with poisonous chemicals by the farmers you will be adding to the toxic load in your body rather than reducing the toxic load. So organic foods, that is, unsprayed foods are especially important during a Detox.

A detox diet alone will not detox you.

Third Step – Detox Formulas

Contrary to much popular belief it takes more than eating nice looking and nice tasting salads for a few days to get those pesky toxins out of your liver or lungs or brain or wherever they are hiding away.

It takes real power to grab these toxin molecules and render them harmless and expel them from the body. It takes special detox herbs, vitamins and minerals. Such a combo is called a Detox Formula.

Fourth Step – Home Detox Techniques

As well as a Detox Diet and a Detox Formula there is little known part of Detox called home detox techniques. I go over 7 of these in the book but let's include one of these super detox techniques here.

Epsom salts Detox

Lying in a comfortably hot bath with a cupful of Epsom salts in the water is not just wonderfully relaxing. It is helping your detox too. The relaxation is helped along by the magnesium in the water and the detox by small amounts of sulphur. Take care not to lose track of time – this is a 15 to 20 minute bath – or you may end up getting so relaxed that you'll have difficulty getting out of the bath – no kidding!

Barry Short

Putting together a tasty diet of salads, fruits, brown rice, soups and a good detox formula and home techniques such as Epsom Salts baths gives you a routine you can use and adapt for 7 days or any other time you wish to detox.

I'd make sure to run it past your family health care professional in case your particular situation such as your health history or medication is an issue.

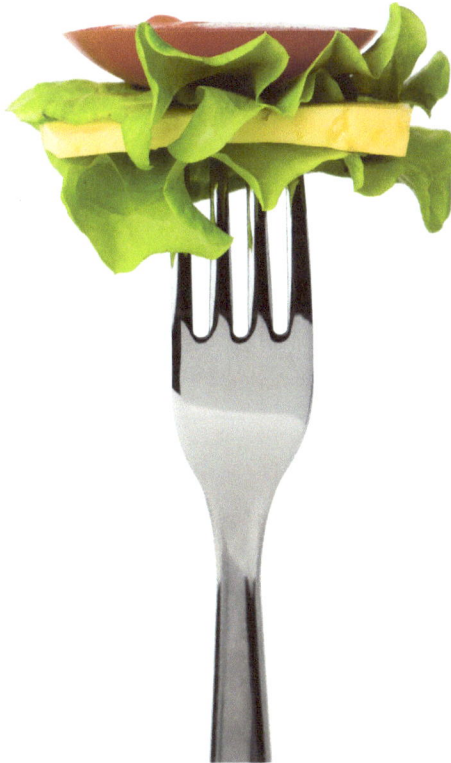

Once you have used this kind of real detox for yourself you'll want to follow it whenever you want to give yourself a break! Detoxing is

Natural Detox Cleanse

like hitting the reboot button on a computer and often leads to increased energy and better sleep. You will then know that your health is in your hands and will have experienced one of the most important methods to improve it.

CHAPTER 10- PELOTHERAPY – HOW TO DETOX

Clay bath, anyone? Sounds luxurious, doesn't it? Pelotherapy, the use of clay for healing, is as old as the hills when it comes to natural medicine. In fact, health spas continue to use clay to this day although you don't need to go to a spa to enjoy the therapeutic effects of clay. You can create clay treatments in your home.

You can find different clays at the market, usually at health food stores, pharmacies and some stores that sell natural supplies. Clay colors come in a wide variety including red, green, blue, pink, yellow and white.

Clays have different mineral compositions according to their color with some clays being more active than others. The most important property that clay has is it great absorptive power; it can remove oil, bacteria, dead skin cells and debris from the skin.

Clay Will Detoxify and Promote Circulation

Clays are used to detoxify the skin and tissues. Clay has the ability to stimulate circulation when it is applied to the skin, which revitalize the skin and underlying tissues.

A general guide to the absorptive power of a clay is the depth of color of a clay. Green and red clays that can be used for body treatments have stronger absorptive powers than light clays, such as pink or white clays, which are more appropriate for facial treatments. In some cases such as for oily skin or acne, a green clay may be used as long as it is not allowed to dry completely on the face.

Natural Detox Cleanse

It is best to choose a clay according to its manufacturer's description and instructions for use since there are so many types of clay from different locations around the world, all with varying mineral compositions and absorptive power.

Deep Cleanse and Detoxify With Clay Based Face and Body Treatments

Clay is used as a main ingredient in many types of face and body treatments such as facial masks, body wraps, baths, foot and hand baths and poultices. Clay facial masks are used for deep cleansing and clarifying treatments for oily and normal skin. For dry or sensitive skins, a clay facial mask may be too drying unless just a small amount of clay is used.

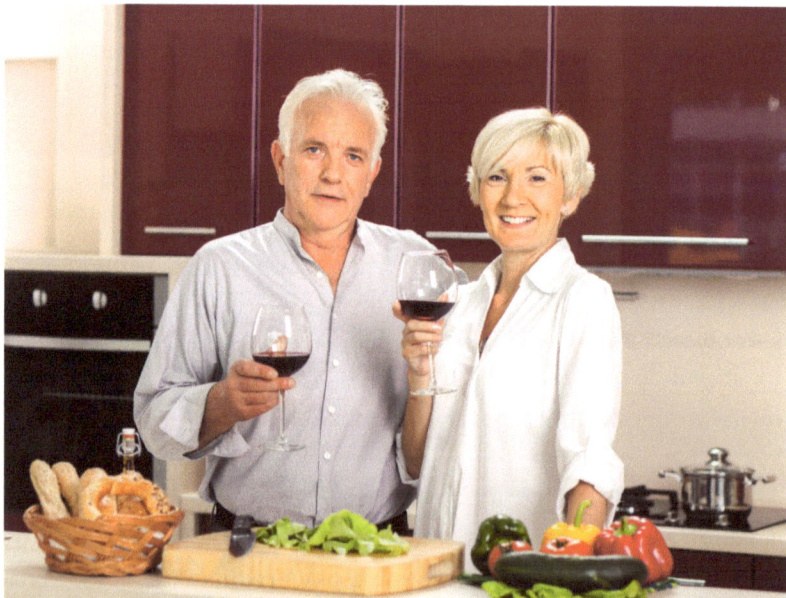

Clay body treatments, such as body wraps and baths, will detoxify the entire body. For medicinal purposes, a clay foot or hand bath can be used to ease some painful conditions, such as arthritis,

Barry Short

because of its detoxifying effects. Clay poultices will ease the sting and itch of insect bites and other minor skin irritations.

Pelotherapy is a versatile natural ingredient for natural healing methods. Clay is so useful for many skin treatments and conditions that it is not surprising that pelotherapy continues to be an important spa treatment for the face and body. Use of clay in the home is an easy way to improve the skin's appearance and to detoxify the body. .

CHAPTER 11- THE BEST DETOX HERB IS?

Herbalists have used Taraxacum Officinale, known as dandelion, as a medicine for centuries. The dandelion root stimulates your digestive glands and your liver. This remarkable herb has many healing properties. Dandelion is the perfect detoxification herb.

The Use of Dandelion in Medicine

Arabian doctors were using dandelion as early as the tenth and twelfth centuries. It has been widely used in the Orient, North America, Australia, Scandinavia, and Europe.

Today, herbalists recommend dandelion as a detoxifying remedy for a wide range of ailments, such as skin complaints and rheumatism. You can use dandelion as a mild laxative, an anti-inflammatory, and a diuretic.

Dandelion combats constipation, weak digestion, and loss of appetite. It is an excellent general tonic for elderly people, and people who are recovering from illness, who prefer a natural remedy. Using dandelion products will add to your feelings of well-being and provide you with an easy to use detoxification method.

How to Use Dandelion in Your Everyday Life

You can purchase many products containing dandelion from your supermarket or health food store. Dandelion teas and coffee are readily available for purchase. You can buy dried dandelion in easy to swallow capsules. Dandelion root powder is in many herbal mixtures that you can obtain from your health food store. Simply stir a spoonful of the herbal mixture into your morning glass of juice.

If you can obtain fresh dandelion leaves, use the leaves to enliven the taste of a salad. Put them in a sandwich instead of lettuce or similar leaves. You can use dried dandelion root to make a refreshing drink or a coffee substitute.

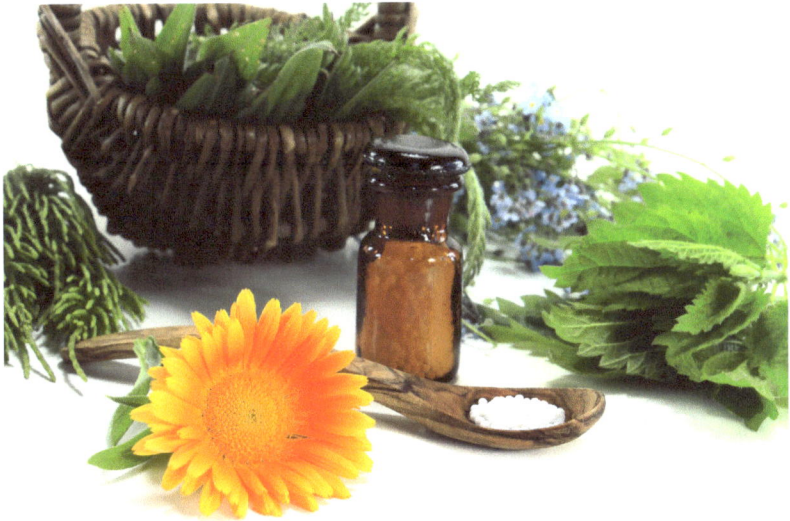

To make your own dandelion drink add one tablespoon of dried dandelion root pieces to a saucepan filled with half a liter of water. Bring this mixture to the boil, turn down the heat, and allow the mixture to simmer for thirty minutes.

Strain the mixture through a tea strainer or a piece of muslin. Add a teaspoon full of honey to sweeten the mixture. Keep the mixture in your refrigerator and use within twenty-four hours.

If you grow your own dandelion, you can make a refreshing homemade coffee substitute. Gather the mature dandelion roots and wash them thoroughly. Dry the roots well, then cut them into small rings. Dry the rings on a drying tray, placed outside in the sunshine. Do not leave the tray out overnight, as it will attract moisture.

Once the pieces are wholly dry, you can roast them in your oven. Set the oven temperature to two hundred degrees centigrade and roast for twenty minutes. Allow to cool. Place the cold roasted rings into either a coffee grinder, or a blender, and reduce to the size of normal coffee granules. Store the granules in an airtight container. Use the granules as a replacement for instant coffee.

You can use the versatile dandelion in many different ways. It makes a perfect detoxification method. Whether you prefer to take it in capsule form, sprinkle it into your juice, make your own drinks from it, or simply eat it in your salads or sandwiches, you will be sure to benefit from its wonderful health giving properties.

CHAPTER 12- LOW CHOLESTEROL MADE EASY

Cholesterol comes in two forms- HDL (good cholesterol) and LDL (bad cholesterol). When people refer to their cholesterol levels, they are usually talking about the overall level.

When the numbers start to rise over 200, that's when doctors raise an eyebrow and recommend lifestyle changes. LDL levels are what contributes to the high end number in lab tests. Depending on the lab or your doctor, the levels for both types may be listed. Lowering cholesterol is important to minimize risk of heart attack and stroke.

Cholesterol may be high due to diet, vitamin deficiency, or genetics. For people suffering from high LDL levels, yet are doing all the 'right' things, medication may be the only option. Once medication is begun, it is often for a lifetime as the cholesterol can rise quickly when medication is discontinued. Lifestyle changes are still beneficial for genetic cholesterol.

To naturally lower cholesterol:

Eat foods known to help increase the HDL levels. Olive oils, canola oil, lean meats. These changes can have significant impact on your LDL levels.

Take garlic supplements. People that take garlic usually see a reduction in their overall cholesterol levels.

Care should be taken to talk with your doctor before using garlic if you are on other medications. Blood thinners, especially - garlic is known to further thin the blood and bleeding from injuries could be dangerous.

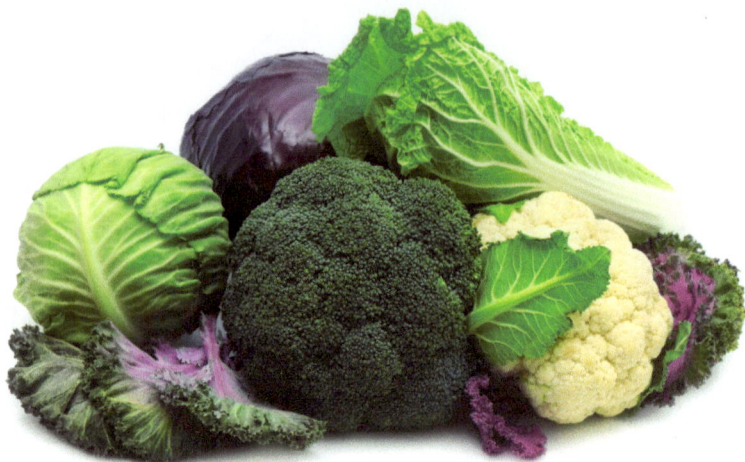

Eat breakfast - grain and oats! Oatmeal is well known for helping reduce cholesterol levels. This grain isn't the only powerhouse out there. Whole grains of all types are good for the body. When combating cholesterol make sure to choose whole grain products.

Quit smoking today. HDL levels begin to rise when a smoker quits. Not only that, but overall health is better.

Have a drink or two. Alcohol, in moderation, is linked with higher HDL levels. Some people drink a small glass of red wine a day. Other alcoholic drinks can contribute to better cholesterol levels, but the sulfites and other chemicals in wine make it a far better choice.

Exercise when possible. Sedentary people tend to carry more weight and higher levels of cholesterol than active folks. Losing weight can help increase the HDL levels and get rid of the LDL. As with smoking, exercise is good for the entire body.

Even a few minutes, several times a day can help. Park further from a store before shopping, use stairs instead of escalators or elevators, and get moving to raise the good and drop the bad.

Get your fish. Omega-3 fatty acids can be found in several types of fish. Wild caught is great, but farmed works well, too. Some doctors prescribe a concentrated form of omega-3s which was developed a few years ago.

For people that avoid seafood or meat products in general, omega-3 fatty acids can be found in some nuts like almonds and in flax seeds. To release the omega-3s in flaxseeds, they must be ground. Just adding whole seeds to foods won't allow you to reap the benefits.

CHAPTER 13- BUST UP THE SUGAR BEFORE YOU DETOX

MYTH: Sugar is harmless.

FALSE

An occasional indulgence is not a problem, but the standard American diet is drowning in sugar! On average, we take in 19 teaspoons of sugar a day; the recommended limit is six teaspoons a day for women, nine for men.

Over time, the high amount of sugar causes weight gain, and is linked to diseases like diabetes. And the energy boost-and-crash cycle leads to cravings for still more sweet stuff, which reinforces the pattern of turning to soft drinks, candy, and other snack foods to reenergize. In fact, a constant high-sugar diet produces changes in brain activity similar to those of a drug addict!

MYTH: Salty snacks like potato chips or pretzels are better than sweet snacks.

FALSE

Starchy foods like potatoes and highly refined grains break down quickly into simple sugars and produce the same chemical reactions in your body. Some of the worst culprits: non-whole-grain bread, pretzels, and pasta.

Barry Short

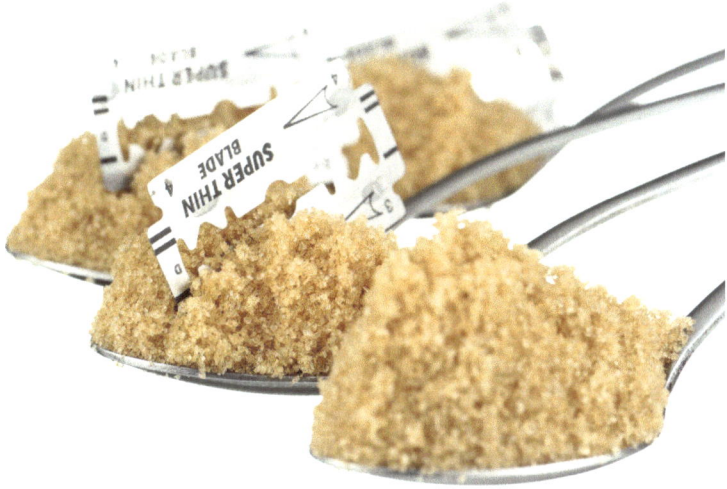

MYTH: Artificially sweetened items are a better choice than products sweetened with sugar.

FALSE

Not really. While artificial sweeteners do have fewer calories, they are still feeding that craving for sweets and keep you on the energy boom-and-bust roller coaster.

MYTH: Natural sweeteners like agave and honey are better than refined white sugars.

FALSE

Sugar is sugar, whether it comes from a bee or a factory! Natural sugars have a slightly higher amount of other nutrients, but they will still bring on the cravings that lead you to overindulge.

MYTH: To break the sugar addiction, you must "detox" by removing ALL sugar from your diet.

Natural Detox Cleanse
FALSE

Sugar detox plans cut out nearly all sugar, including all fruits and some of the sweeter veggies like peas and carrots. This is a sudden and drastic change, and can work in the short run but is hard to maintain. And if anything, the swings between overindulgence and strict sugar-fasting will actually make your cravings stronger.

MYTH: Once you are addicted to the sweet stuff, there's nothing you can do about it--you are hooked for life.

FALSE

You CAN wean yourself off a diet heavy in simple sugars! The secret is to take small steps rather than sudden dramatic change. Here are some steps to take:

-- Cut out one sweet indulgence each week rather than all at once. Start by eliminating dessert from either lunch or dinner, or skipping that 3 PM chocolate bar.

-- Drink more water. Most of the time what feels like an overwhelming need for a sugary soft drink is just simple thirst.

-- Read labels. In addition to the large amounts of in our foods that are labelled as such, plenty sneaks in under different descriptions. Watch out for terms like "high fructose corn syrup", "cane syrup", or "dextrose", which all mean "sugar" under a different name.

-- Get out and move! In addition to being great for your body and your stress levels, exercise tends to increase the body's cravings for healthier foods, which in turn will help develop your taste for them.

Barry Short

-- <u>When you do indulge your sweet</u> tooth with fruits and other naturally sweet products. They have fiber and other nutrients that slow the breaking down process, so the sugar dump into the bloodstream is not as fast. If you have to have chocolate, choose a high quality dark chocolate and eat just a little.

--<u>Try to make desserts</u> an occasional treat rather than a daily necessity. If you tend to have a nightly bowl of ice cream before bed, try substituting a glass of low fat or skim milk, sipped slowly.

Small changes over time will add up! And as you take in fewer sweets, your taste for the super sugary stuff will wane as well, reducing your cravings.

ABOUT THE AUTHOR

Barry Short was introduced to the detox process by his wife and ever since he experienced the benefits himself, he has been sharing the information with everyone that he can. He has written quite a number of books and all of them are focused on various health topics.

The detox diet is his favorite niche however and he focuses on various types in his latest book. Barry leaves the reader to determine whether or not they will embrace the detox diet at the end of the day.